SOMATIC EXERCISE FOR WEIGHT LOSS

Beginners guide to reduce belly fat, eliminate anxiety, stress, and improve emotional balance

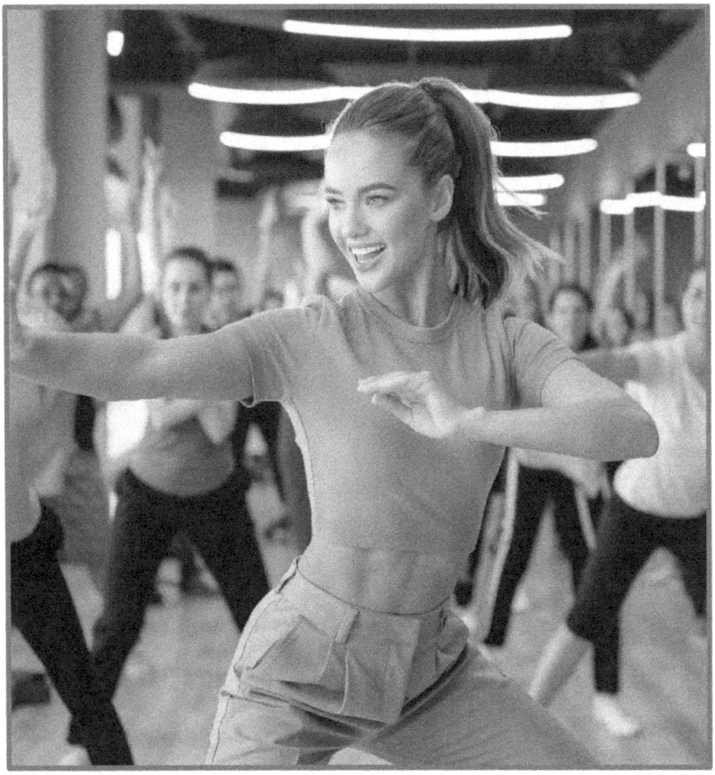

HARRY LAVELLE

TABLE OF CONTENT

TABLE OF CONTENT 3

INTRODUCTION 7

PART I: BUILDING THE FOUNDATION FOR SOMATIC WEIGHT LOSS 16

CHAPTER 1: ESSENTIAL IDEAS OF SOMATIC EXERCISE FOR LOSING WEIGHT 17

Understanding Your Body's Signals to Improve Body Awareness 17

PART II: YOUR PRACTICAL GUIDE TO SOMATIC EXERCISES FOR WEIGHT LOSS 24

The Grounded Warrior (Mountain Pose with Diaphragmatic Breathing) 25

The Dancing Tree (Tree Pose with Gentle Swaying) 29

The Flowing River (Cat-Cow Pose) 31

The Serene Swan (Modified Cobra Pose) 33

The Peaceful Ocean (Constructive Rest Pose) 35

CHAPTER 2: WARMING UP AND FOUNDATIONAL SOMATIC EXERCISES 37

Warming Up Essentials: Getting Your Body Ready for Somatic Exercise 37

Basic Somatic Activities: Increasing Stability and Core Strength 39

Including Mindfulness in Your Work: Developing Body Consciousness 40

CHAPTER 3: SPECIFIC SOMATIC EXERCISES FOR ROBUST WEIGHT LOSS 43

Sculpting Your Midsection and Increasing Metabolism with Core Strengthening 43

Taking Care of Particular Issues: Back Pain, Tight Hips, and Other Exercises 46

Developing a Customized Somatic Exercise Program: Taking Your Needs Into Account 50

CHAPTER 4: MINDFUL MOVEMENT AND RELAXATION FOR WEIGHT MANAGEMENT 57

Stress Reduction Techniques: Guided Meditations and Breath work 57

Creating Your Personalized Stress-Reduction Sanctuary 59

Gentle Yoga-Inspired Flows: Promoting Relaxation and Restoration... 61

Mindful Eating Practices: Cultivating a Healthy Relationship with Food 66

PART III: SUPPORTING YOUR WEIGHT LOSS JOURNEY WITH SOMATIC PRACTICES.................... 69

CHAPTER 5: NUTRITION AND SOMATIC EXERCISE: A HOLISTIC APPROACH 69

Eating for Energy and Weight Loss: The Somatic Nutrition Principles 69

Mindful Eating in Practice: Tips and Techniques for Success 73

Sample Meal Plans and Recipes: Delicious and Nourishing Options 77

CHAPTER 6: LIFESTYLE HABITS FOR LONG-TERM WEIGHT MANAGEMENT SUCCESS........................... 81

Sleep: The Essential Ingredient for Weight Loss and Overall Health.. 81

The Metabolic Symphony: Energy Expenditure and Glucose Regulation 83

Stress Management: Strategies for Reducing Stress and Emotional Eating 85

Creating a Supportive Environment: Building a Foundation for Success 89

PART IV: INSPIRATION AND RESOURCES 93

CHAPTER 7: SUCCESS STORIES: REAL PEOPLE, REAL TRANSFORMATIONS 93

Inspiring Stories of Weight Loss through Somatic Exercise: Finding Motivation 93

Overcoming Challenges and Plateaus: Lessons from Others' Journeys 95

CONCLUSION 99

INTRODUCTION

Are you tired of battling stubborn belly fat that seems impervious to traditional diet and exercise? Do you find yourself constantly wrestling with anxiety and stress, struggling to maintain emotional balance in your daily life? If so, you're not alone. Millions of people face these interconnected challenges, often feeling frustrated and overwhelmed. But what if there was a holistic approach that could address both your physical and emotional well-being simultaneously?

Flora wasn't lazy; she was trapped. A gnawing exhaustion had settled into her bones, a weight far heavier than the extra pounds she carried. Diets had failed her, workouts had felt impossible, and a deep frustration had festered within. Her reflection mocked her, her energy dwindled, and life's vibrancy seemed out of reach.

One day, a whisper of hope emerged – my book, "Somatic Exercises for Weight Loss." Flora was skeptical, but desperation nudged her toward its pages. As she delved into the concept of somatic movement – exercises designed to reconnect mind and body – a flicker of curiosity ignited.

She began tentatively, exploring gentle movements that felt more like dance than drudgery. Slowly, something shifted. The exercises weren't just about burning calories; they were about awakening her body's wisdom, tuning into its signals, and honoring its needs.

Weeks turned into months. The weight began to melt away, not through grueling workouts, but through joyful movement. Flora's energy surged, her confidence blossomed, and a newfound radiance illuminated her eyes.

Her transformation wasn't just physical; it was a reawakening of her spirit. The exercises had unlocked a wellspring of vitality she never knew existed. The woman who had once felt trapped in her own body was now free – free to move, free to live, free to thrive.

If you're tired of battling your body, if diets and workouts have left you feeling defeated, it's time for a new approach. "Somatic Exercises for Weight Loss" isn't just another fitness fad; it's a journey of self-discovery, a path toward sustainable transformation.

In these pages, you'll find the tools to reconnect with your body's innate wisdom, to ignite your metabolism, and to release the weight that's been holding you back – both physically and emotionally.

But don't just take my word for it. Flora's story is one of many. Countless others have found freedom and joy through the power of somatic movement. This isn't about quick fixes; it's about lasting change.

Don't wait another day to reclaim your vitality. Your body is a masterpiece waiting to be unveiled. Turn the page, and let the journey begin.

WHAT IS SOMATIC EXERCISE?

Somatic exercise is a kind of attentive, gentle movement that focuses on the body's internal experience. In contrast to conventional exercise regimens that emphasize outward form and repetition, somatic exercises foster an in-depth awareness of your body's internal movements and sensations. Thomas Hanna created Clinical Somatic Education in the 1970s to treat mobility impairments and chronic pain. This approach is based on his work.

Somatic exercise helps relieve tension, improve posture, and heighten general body awareness by reestablishing the connection between your brain and your muscles and neurological system. Its inward emphasis makes yoga an effective tool for stress, anxiety, and emotional well-being management in addition to physical change.

BENEFITS SOMATIC EXERCISE'S FOR EMOTIONAL AND WEIGHT LOSS

The twin benefits of somatic exercise for the body and mind are what make it so beautiful. Somatic exercises are effective for weight reduction, especially for abdominal fat that is hard to lose. They do this by:

1. Correcting alignment and posture, which may quickly make you seem smaller

2. Improving body awareness and muscular tone, which results in more effective movement

3. Decreased production of cortisol, which is connected to the accumulation of fat in the abdomen, due to stress

4. Improving whole body functioning, which facilitates and enhances the effectiveness of various types of exercise

However, THE ADVANTAGES go much beyond bodily modifications. A potent technique for emotional and mental wellness is somatic exercise, which aids in:

1. Reduce anxiety by encouraging bodily awareness and serenity.

2. Decrease tension by using breathing and mindful movement practices

Enhance emotional equilibrium by cultivating a more robust mind-body link

4. As you have more control over your body and emotions, increase your self-confidence.

You will come across first-hand accounts and testimonies from people who have personally experienced these life-changing impacts throughout this book.

HOW TO UTILIZE THIS MANUAL

This book aims to guide you from a basic grasp of somatic exercise to a complete integration of it into your everyday routine. Here's what to anticipate:

1. An extensive examination of the philosophy, science, and history of somatic exercise

2. Detailed directions for fundamental somatic routines and exercises

3. Detailed instructions on how to use somatic exercise to manage emotions, reduce stress, and lose weight

4. Useful advice for developing a long-lasting habit of somatic exercise

5. Case studies and real-world success stories

6. Extra materials to help you continue your practice

I want you to approach this book with an open mind and a readiness to experiment with new bodily experiences so that you may get the most out of it. Go slowly through each chapter, repeating the exercises often and noting your feelings as you go. Keep in mind that somatic exercise is about the internal experience, so don't force or strain yourself. Move at your own speed and pay attention to your body.

Remind yourself that consistency is essential as you set out on your road. Over time, even a short daily practice session might provide noticeable outcomes. Have patience with yourself and acknowledge your little accomplishments as you go.

Are you prepared to experience the life-changing potential of somatic training? Let's start your journey towards a more balanced emotional life, a smaller waist, and a calmer mind by turning the page. Now is the time to begin your path to comprehensive well-being!

PART I: BUILDING THE FOUNDATION FOR SOMATIC WEIGHT LOSS

CHAPTER 1: ESSENTIAL IDEAS OF SOMATIC EXERCISE FOR LOSING WEIGHT

Understanding Your Body's Signals to Improve Body Awareness

Body awareness is a symphony of feelings that are sometimes lost in the din of contemporary life. It is the secret language of our physical body. Consider your body as a finely tuned instrument that is continuously communicating its requirements and states. These signals, which range from the little flutter in your stomach before making an important choice to the warmth that fills your chest during happy times, comprise a complex tapestry of information that is just waiting to be unraveled.

It's similar to learning to hear whispers in a loud setting to cultivate this sensitivity. It takes time, effort, and a readiness to calm the mind. Deeper exploration of this technique will provide a multitude of insights.

Unrecognized stress may be indicated by the stiffness in your shoulders, and a sudden urge for greens may indicate a nutritional deficiency.

There is more to this self-discovery path than just physical experiences. Developing body awareness may help you become more intuitive, develop emotional intelligence, and even strengthen your bonds with others. You're not only listening to a group of cells and processes when you tune into your body's wisdom; rather, you're accessing a long-forgotten, intrinsic intellect that may direct you toward better health, joy, and harmony.

Thus, stop, inhale deeply, and pay attention. What secrets does your body now reveal to you?

Using Your Muscles with Intention and Awareness during Mindful Movement

A mindful movement is a dance between the body and the mind, a symphony in which every muscle fiber has a purposeful, graceful role to perform. Consider your body as a well-tuned instrument, with every action serving as a note in an intricate song of awareness and purpose.

You are exploring the terrain of your physical form while you do this, rather than merely working out. As you stretch, pay attention to the minute interactions between your muscles: the whisper of tendons adapting, the delicate stretching of fibers. You're creating a clear mental image of your inner workings with every movement.

This has nothing to do with setting a personal record or mastering a stance. It's about living in the poetry of motion to the fullest. Observe how your breathing matches your motions and how your weight changes as you maintain balance. Take note of the series of little adaptations your body makes to itself with every little shift in posture.

By moving mindfully, you may turn ordinary activities into self-discovering ones. A stroll turns into a meditation on the precise synchronization of the legs and core. A weightlifting exercise turns into a study of strength and limits.

By bringing purpose and awareness into your physical activities, you're not simply strengthening your muscles; you're developing a stronger connection between your body and mind and opening up new avenues for self-knowledge and well-being.

<u>Breath work</u>: Using Your Breath's Power to Lose Weight

Breath work is a secret weapon in your health toolbox that is often disregarded when it comes to losing weight. Think of your breath as a gentle but powerful force that may activate your body's natural processes that burn fat. When used properly, this age-old method may transform your weight reduction journey into a symphony of physiological changes.

You'll learn about breath work's many effects as you explore it. Breathing deeply and rhythmically activates your vague nerve, which sets off a series of events that reduce cortisol levels, the stress hormone that is known to encourage abdominal fat that won't go away. This deliberate breathing simultaneously increases oxygen flow, fanning the flames of your metabolism like a bellows to a flame.

However, breathwork's power goes beyond biology. It turns into a tool for awareness, guiding you through the emotional terrain of eating. Your connection with food may be completely changed by taking those deliberate breaths during the times of silence before meals. You will become more sensitive to hunger signals naturally and less likely to overeat while under stress.

Furthermore, breathing exercises such as "breath of fire" or "alternating nostril breathing" may stimulate your body and provide energy for exercise without giving you the jittery side effects of coffee. By becoming proficient in these methods, you will not only shed pounds but also acquire a lifetime ability to maintain your whole health.

Embodiment: Fostering a Close Bond with Your Physical Form

Being fully aware of your physical self while inhabiting it is the art of embodiment, which goes beyond simple survival to include the whole range of physical experience. Think of your body as a complex environment that you explore with every breath and movement, rather than as a vessel that you inhabit.

Awakening your senses is the first step on your path towards embodiment. Feel the softness of the air on your skin, the little movement of your muscles as you correct your alignment, and the resounding pounding of your heart in your chest. Every feeling opens a doorway to a more profound awareness of oneself.

You are going to learn the secret language of your body as you develop this relationship. A flutter in your stomach might indicate intuitive understanding, while stiffness in your shoulders could be a hint of unrecognized tension. These bodily signals become insightful information via embodiment, influencing your choices and raising your emotional intelligence.

Movement is also redefined by embodiment. A stroll turns into a well-coordinated symphony, with every stride an expression of your body's potential. You'll discover a new level of presence in silence, sensing the life force that flows through you even in sleep.

The goal of this exercise is to embrace the unique tale that your body has to tell, not to achieve perfection. When you live completely from your body, you access a rich reservoir of knowledge, inspiration, and energy that has the power to transform every area of your life.

PART II: YOUR PRACTICAL GUIDE TO SOMATIC EXERCISES FOR WEIGHT LOSS

The Grounded Warrior (Mountain Pose with Diaphragmatic Breathing)

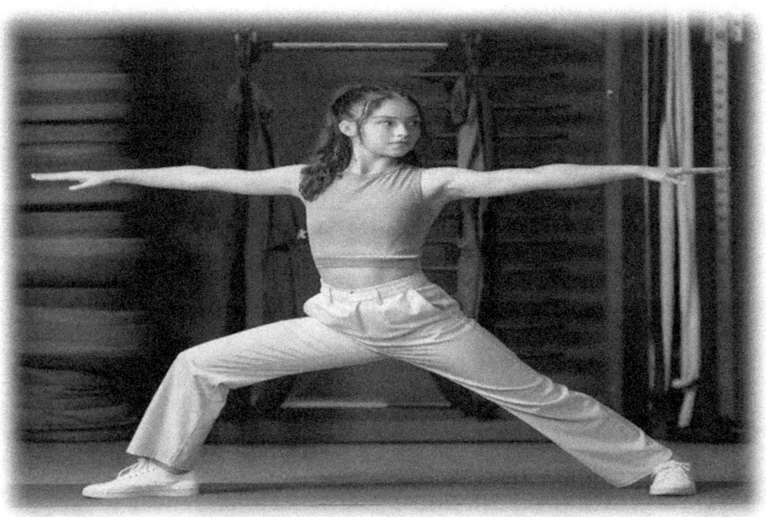

Definition: Mountain Pose, is a foundational pose in yoga that emphasizes proper alignment and posture. When combined with diaphragmatic breathing (belly breathing), it becomes a powerful tool for grounding, centering, and calming the nervous system.

Instructions: Stand tall with your feet hip-width apart. Ground down through your feet, feeling the connection to the earth. Engage your leg muscles, lifting your kneecaps slightly. Lengthen your spine, relax your shoulders, and gently tuck your tailbone. Inhale deeply, allowing your belly to expand fully. Exhale slowly, drawing your navel towards your spine.

Benefits:

Improved Posture: Mountain Pose promotes proper alignment of the spine, shoulders, and hips, which can help alleviate back pain and improve overall posture.

Core Strength: Engaging the leg muscles and core helps to strengthen these areas, leading to a more stable and supported posture.

Stress Reduction: Diaphragmatic breathing activates the parasympathetic nervous system, promoting relaxation and reducing stress. This can be particularly beneficial for weight loss, as stress is often a trigger for unhealthy eating habits.

Enhanced Body Awareness: By focusing on the sensations within your body, you develop a greater sense of proprioception and body awareness, which can translate to more mindful movement in other activities.

Improved Digestion: The diaphragmatic breathing component of this exercise massages the abdominal organs and can aid in digestion.

Sets and Reps: Hold the pose for 5-10 breaths, repeating 3-5 times.

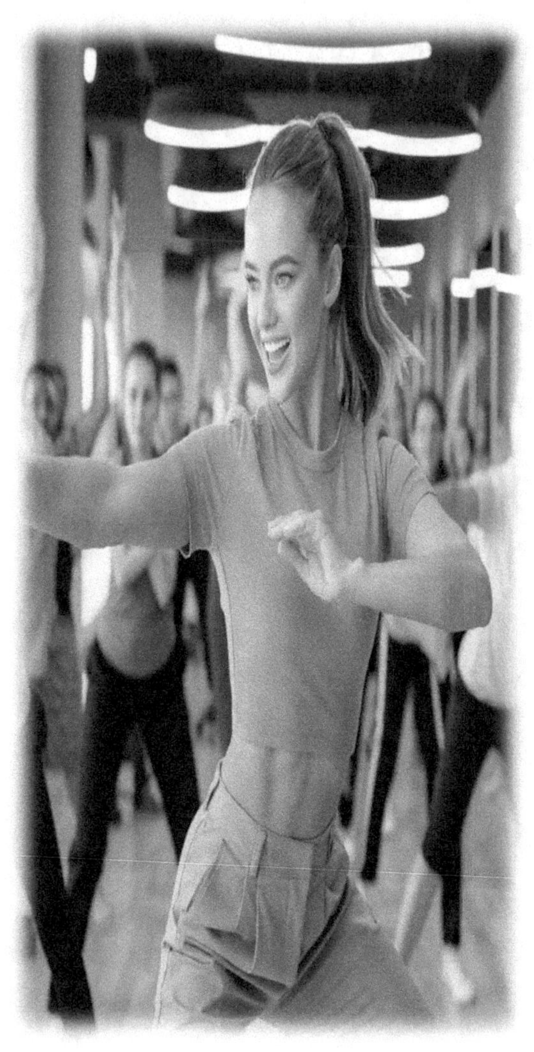

The Dancing Tree (Tree Pose with Gentle Swaying)

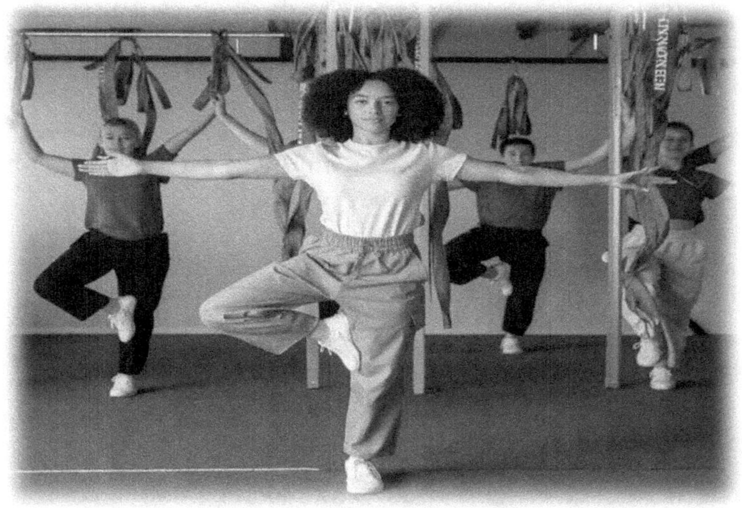

Definition: Tree Pose, is a balancing pose that requires focus, concentration, and strength. By incorporating gentle swaying, you engage your core muscles and challenge your balance while cultivating a sense of playfulness and freedom.

Instructions: Stand on one leg, bending the opposite knee and placing the sole of your foot on your inner thigh or calf. Avoid placing your foot directly on your knee joint. Find your balance, fixing your gaze on a steady point in front of you. Gently sway your body from side to side, like a tree in the breeze. Focus on your breath and the sensations in your body.

Benefits:

Enhanced Balance: This pose challenges your balance and proprioception, helping to improve coordination and stability.

Leg and Core Strength: Balancing on one leg engages the muscles of the standing leg and core, strengthening these areas.

Improved Concentration: Maintaining your balance requires focus and concentration, which can have positive effects on mental clarity and focus.

Playfulness and Joy: The gentle swaying motion adds an element of playfulness to the pose, helping to release tension and cultivate a sense of joy in movement.

Sets and Reps: Hold the pose on each side for 5-10 breaths, repeating 2-3 times.

The Flowing River (Cat-Cow Pose)

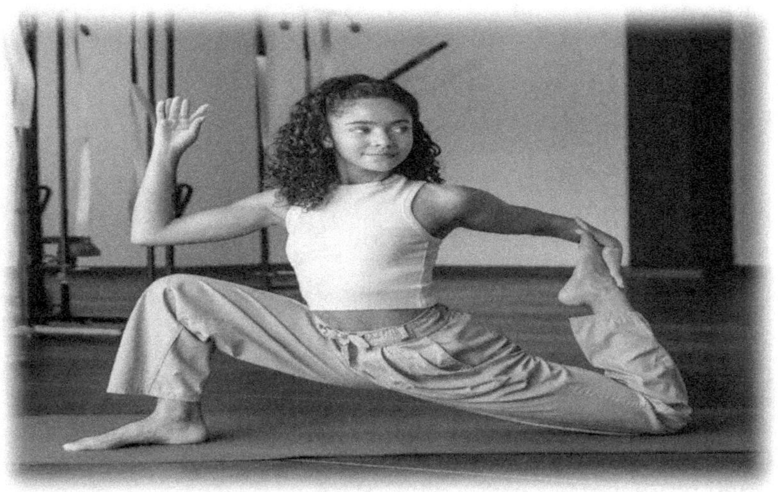

Definition: Cat-Cow Pose, is a gentle spinal movement that combines flexion (rounding of the spine) and extension (arching of the spine). This rhythmic movement can help to improve spinal mobility, release tension in the back and neck, and promote relaxation.

Instructions: Start on your hands and knees, aligning your wrists under your shoulders and your knees under your hips. Inhale, arching your back like a cat and lifting your chin. Exhale, rounding your spine like a cow and tucking your chin. Repeat, syncing your movement with your breath.

Benefits:

Increased Spinal Flexibility: The flowing movement between flexion and extension helps to improve spinal mobility and flexibility, reducing stiffness and discomfort.

Abdominal Massage: The gentle movement of the spine massages the abdominal organs, which can aid in digestion and promote healthy gut function.

Stress Relief: The rhythmic movement and focus on breath can have a calming effect on the nervous system, reducing stress and anxiety.

Back Pain Relief: By mobilizing the spine and releasing tension in the back muscles, Cat-Cow Pose can help to alleviate back pain.

Sets and Reps: Flow through 5-10 rounds, focusing on the connection between your breath and movement.

The Serene Swan (Modified Cobra Pose)

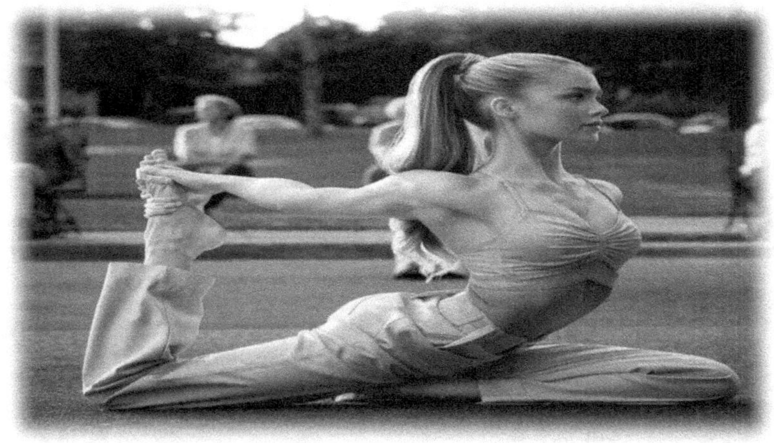

Definition: Modified Cobra Pose, is a gentle backbend that opens the chest, stretches the spine, and strengthens the back muscles. This pose is a gentler variation of the full Cobra Pose (Bhujangasana) and is often more accessible for beginners.

Instructions: Lie on your stomach, placing your hands under your shoulders with your elbows close to your body. Inhale, lifting your chest and head while keeping your pelvis grounded. Keep your elbows bent and your neck long. Gaze forward or slightly upward. Exhale, gently lowering back down.

Benefits:

Spinal Stretch and Strength: The backbend motion stretches the front of the body and strengthens the muscles of the back and spine.

Chest and Shoulder Opening: The pose opens the chest and shoulders, counteracting the effects of slouching and promoting better posture. This can also help to improve breathing capacity.

Stress Relief: Backbends like Cobra Pose are known to have a stimulating effect on the nervous system, which can help to relieve stress and improve mood.

Emotional Release: The opening of the chest can also facilitate emotional release, helping to reduce anxiety and tension.

Sets and Reps: Hold the pose for 5-10 breaths, repeating 3-5 times.

The Peaceful Ocean (Constructive Rest Pose)

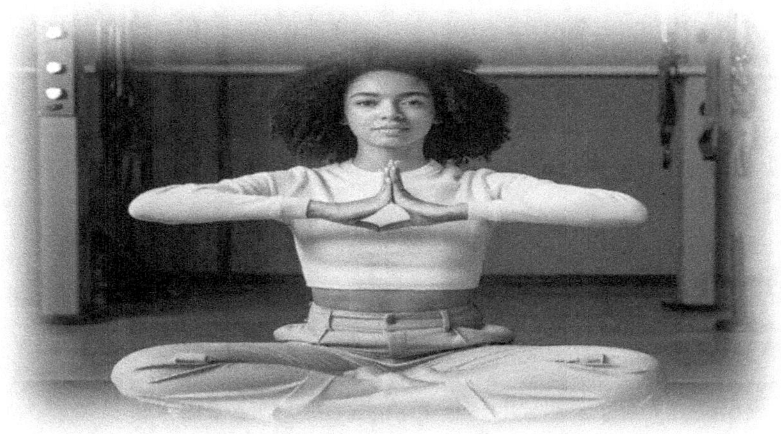

Definition: Constructive Rest Pose is a restorative yoga pose that involves lying on your back with your knees bent and feet flat on the floor. This position encourages deep relaxation, release of tension, and a sense of grounding.

Instructions: Lie on your back with your knees bent and feet flat on the floor. Place a small pillow or folded blanket under your head for support. Rest your arms by your sides, palms facing up. Close your eyes and allow your body to fully relax.

Benefits:

Deep Relaxation: This pose promotes deep relaxation of the muscles and nervous system, helping to reduce stress and fatigue.

Improved Digestion: The gentle pressure on the abdomen can aid in digestion and relieve bloating.

Mindfulness and Body Awareness: By focusing on your breath and the sensations in your body, you cultivate mindfulness and a deeper connection with yourself.

Stress Reduction: The restorative nature of this pose can help to reduce cortisol levels (the stress hormone) and promote a sense of calm.

Sets and Reps: Rest in this pose for 5-10 minutes, focusing on your breath and allowing your body to melt into the floor.

CHAPTER 2: WARMING UP AND FOUNDATIONAL SOMATIC EXERCISES

Warming Up Essentials: Getting Your Body Ready for Somatic Exercise

Think of your body as a well-tuned instrument that is just ready to be stimulated. Warming up before somatic activity is more than simply a preamble; it's a ritual that shifts consciousness and helps one get from stillness to action. Imagine every muscle fiber waking up as you start, much like a symphony orchestra getting ready for a big show.

Begin with mild oscillations, letting your body gently rock back and forth. Sensate the minute changes in weight to activate your body's natural sense of position, or proprioception. Then, move your joints, little and large, from your toes to your neck, as if you were oiling a complicated machinery. Your system experiences awareness tremors with every small spin.

Your silent companion in this preparatory dance is breath work. Breathe deeply and rhythmically to oxygenate your tissues and fuel your metabolism. Visualize life extending to each and every cell as you inhale, and release any remaining tension as you exhale.

Expand your range of motion gradually, as if you were a flower softly unfolding its petals. Include dynamic stretches that resemble the motions of the activity you will be doing, preparing your brain to communicate with your muscles effectively.

This warm-up is more than simply physical; it's also a mental practice that establishes goals for the next somatic adventure. By the conclusion, you're embodied, present, and prepared for a deep study of movement, not simply for physical activity.

Basic Somatic Activities: Increasing Stability and Core Strength

Basic somatic exercises weave a tapestry of power from your inner core and are the cornerstone of physical awareness and control. Think of your core as a dynamic powerhouse that radiates stability and energy outward rather than merely being a collection of muscles.

These are not your typical crunches or planks. Rather, they encourage you to investigate delicate, nuanced motions that reawaken slumbering neuronal networks. Imagine yourself rolling through your spine with mild pelvic tilts, each vertebra articulating as you do so. As you advance, the cat-cow flow transforms into a wave of feeling, with every movement acting as a whisper of mind and body connection.

From a straightforward opposing arm-leg extension, the bird-dog exercise develops into a proprioception and balance study. Observe the little changes your body makes to stay balanced; every tremble is an indication that your stabilizer muscles are waking up.

Breath becomes your anchor while working with somatic core exercises. In addition to taking deep breaths, the diaphragmatic breathing exercise involves massaging your internal organs, feeling your ribcage expand in three dimensions, and releasing tension in your deep abdominal muscles in a rhythmic manner.

These fundamental exercises provide the framework for a body that moves with strength, elegance, and intention—turning common motions into manifestations of embodied strength.

Including Mindfulness in Your Work: Developing Body Consciousness

Within the context of somatic practice, mindfulness serves as a transformational prism through which every movement becomes an in-depth investigation of the self. Visualize your awareness as a calm river that permeates every muscle and cell in your body, bringing to light experiences that are often missed by the ordinary conscious mind.

Start by establishing your grounding in the here and now. Sensate the feel of the air on your skin and the feel of the floor underneath you. Just seeing things turns into an anchor that keeps you in the present moment.

Explore the geography of your body with every breath. Take note of your abdomen's delicate rise and fall as well as the modest expansion of your ribcage. Develop a feeling of inquiry as you go. How does your weight change? Can you sense how your muscles work together and how your body modifies itself slightly to stay balanced?

Accept every feeling without passing judgment. A little constriction transforms into an opportunity for growth rather than a weakness. Easy times are thoroughly enjoyed, which produces a positive feedback loop that motivates further practice.

As you become more conscious, you could get unexpected insights. Maybe you hunch your shoulders or tighten your teeth out of habit. Both on and off the mat, these insights provide chances for release and realignment.

You may take your somatic practice beyond simple physical activity by including awareness. It turns into a quest for self-awareness and a dynamic meditation that strengthens the connection between the body and the mind.

CHAPTER 3: SPECIFIC SOMATIC EXERCISES FOR ROBUST WEIGHT LOSS

Sculpting Your Midsection and Increasing Metabolism with Core Strengthening

Achieving washboard abs is not the only goal of core strengthening; it's also a trip to discover your body's secret powers. Think of your core as a dynamic, three-dimensional cylinder that includes your deep internal muscles, pelvic floor, lower back, and abdominals.

While doing core exercises, picture each movement as a tool used by a sculptor, chipping away at your stomach and fueling your metabolic fire at the same time. When executed mindfully, the simple plank transforms into a full-body stability meditation. Your muscles will tremble slightly as they cooperate to maintain your alignment.

Rotational exercises, like as Russian twists, are great for improving functional strength for daily activities, igniting your internal fire, and targeting love handles. They also increase lymphatic drainage. Visualize expelling poisons and stagnated energy from your organs as you twist.

However, when you include breathing into your daily practice, the true magic occurs. When doing exercises like hollow body holds, take deep, diaphragmatic breaths to massage your internal organs, improve circulation, and enhance your workout.

By strengthening your core, you're laying the groundwork for improved posture, less back discomfort, and an efficient metabolism that lasts long after your exercise. You're not only creating a slimmer silhouette.

Whole-Body Flows: Increasing Dexterity, Strength, and Burning Fat

Whole-body flows are the perfect example of how to take a holistic approach to improving your body's strength, flexibility, and ability to burn fat. Imagine switching between exercises with ease, feeling every muscle contract and stretch, every sinew growing. Full-body flows are dynamic sequences that integrate numerous muscle groups, resulting in a harmonic synergy that enhances your fitness results. They are more than simply exercises.

You move fluidly through these flows, from postures that strengthen your core to stretches that increase your flexibility to high-intensity exercises that burn fat. Every flow is a choreography of movements designed to test your physical and mental faculties while maintaining your motivation and interest.

Including full-body flows in your exercise routine allows you to take advantage of a multidimensional strategy that enhances your performance. By guaranteeing that every muscle is engaged, these fluxes lower the chance of injury and encourage balanced muscular growth. Additionally, the constant moving between workouts maintains a raised heart rate, which improves cardiovascular health and speeds up fat loss.

Learn how full-body flows may alter your life. Take up an exercise regimen that will not only tone your body but also lift your mood and make you stronger, more flexible, and full of energy. Encountering the elegant, powerful movements of full-body flows is the first step towards becoming a more fit and well-er person.

Taking Care of Particular Issues: Back Pain, Tight Hips, and Other Exercises

Are you sick of your back hurting all the time? Do tense hips make it difficult for you to move and make you unhappy? It's time to recover your vigor and escape the bonds of discomfort. Your secret to a life of improved mobility, less pain, and regenerated vitality is this all-inclusive handbook. We'll explore the nuances of tight hips and back discomfort, giving you a wealth of exercises that specifically address these issues as well as insightful analysis and pointers to help you obtain the best possible results.

Recognizing Back Pain: Exposing the Fundamental Causes

Back discomfort is a common condition that may be caused by a number of things, such as:

• **Muscle Strain:** Pain and stiffness may result from overstretching, poor posture, and repeated motions that strain the muscles that support your spine.

• **Disc Issues:** Compressing nerves due to herniated or bulging discs may cause intense, stabbing pain.

• **Arthritis:** Chronic pain and inflammation may be caused by degenerative changes in the spine's joints.

• **Spinal Stenosis:** When the spinal canal narrows, pressure is applied to the nerves, causing pain, numbness, and weakness.

Cracking Tight Hips: A More Detailed Look

Back discomfort and tight hips often go hand in hand. The following factors may cause the muscles that surround your hip joint to become tight and restricted: ● Sedentary Lifestyle: Extended periods of sitting can shorten and tighten the hip flexor muscles, which can cause pain and restricted movement.

● **Muscle Imbalance:** Your posture and movement patterns may be impacted by an imbalance caused by tight hip flexors and weak gluteal muscles.

● **Overuse or Injury:** Inflammation and stiffness in the hip joint may result from overuse or injury.

Your Customized Workout Schedule: Tailored Remedies for Maximum Solace

Here is a carefully chosen list of exercises meant to help with your particular issues:

• **Cat-Cow Pose:** This mild yoga position eases stiffness and increases flexibility by warming up and mobilizing your spine.

• **Bird Dog:** Enhance your stability and balance by strengthening your back and core muscles.

• **Bridge:** To relieve strain on your lower back and encourage correct alignment, contract your hamstrings and glutes.

• **Knee-to-Chest Stretch**: This stretch helps to relax and relieve discomfort by releasing tension in your hips and lower back.

• **Pelvic tilts**: These exercises may help reduce back discomfort by strengthening your core and improving pelvic stability.

Tight Hips? Try Pigeon Pose, a deep hip opener that stretches your glutes, piriformis, and hip flexors to release tension and increase flexibility.

• **Figure Four Stretch:** Increase your range of motion by releasing tightness in your glutes and hips.

Stretch your tight hip flexors, since they may be a contributing factor to back discomfort and restricted range of motion.

● **Foam Rolling:** To promote relaxation and ease tension, roll a foam roller over the tight muscles in your glutes and hips.

● **Butterfly Stretch:** To increase flexibility and lessen hip stiffness, gently stretch the muscles in your inner thighs and groin.

Developing a Customized Somatic Exercise Program: Taking Your Needs Into Account

Are you longing for an exercise regimen that explores the deep relationship between mind and body and goes beyond simple physicality? You just need to look at the changing field of somatic movement. This all-inclusive manual will enable you to design a customized somatic exercise program that meets your individual goals and objectives, opening up a world of improved body awareness, less discomfort, and renewed vigor.

Revealing the Secret Nature of Somatic Motion

A comprehensive approach to fitness, somatic movement places a focus on careful awareness of your body's internal sensations. Somatic activities help you become more aware of your movement patterns and habits by helping you to tune into your body's subtle messages, in contrast to standard exercises that only concentrate on external objectives. You may detect and release chronic tension, correct posture, and move more easily and fluidly by practicing this elevated awareness.

The Influence of Customization

The versatility of somatic movement is among its most amazing features. There is no one-size-fits-all method; rather, you are free to design a practice that suits your own requirements, tastes, and objectives. Somatic exercises may be customized to match your unique needs, whether it pain alleviation, stress reduction, or improved sports performance.

How to Create a Somatic Retreat

This is a step-by-step tutorial to help you design your own somatic exercise regimen:

1. Self-Evaluation Start by focusing on the particular terrain of your body. Which parts feel constrained or tight? Exist any nagging aches or pains? Which motions are the most pleasurable and natural?

2. Investigate Diverse Modalities: Somatic movement is a vast tapestry of techniques, each with a unique character. Investigate several modalities to find what speaks to you: Feldenkrais, Alexander Technique, Body-Mind Centering, Hanna Somatic.

3. **Seek Guidance:** Take into account consulting with a licensed somatic therapist or instructor. Their knowledge may assist you in improving your methods, taking care of certain issues, and realizing the full potential of your practice.

4. **Develop Mindfulness:** One mindful practice is somatic movement. Observe your body's feelings carefully as you move, noting any regions of ease or stress. Take deep breaths and let your motions come naturally to you.

5. Begin Little: Start with brief, concentrated sessions and work your way up in length and intensity as your body adjusts. Recall that somatic movement is about recognizing your body's knowledge and listening to it rather than pushing yourself over your comfort zone.

6. Appreciate Variety: Don't be scared to try out new routines and workouts. In addition to pushing your body in novel and surprising ways, variety makes your exercise interesting and lively.

7. Incorporate into Everyday Life: Somatic movement isn't limited to set exercise periods. Incorporate posture corrections, breathing techniques, and easy stretches into your everyday practice to promote conscious movement.

Examples of Somatic Activities

Some somatic exercises that you might include in your program are as follows:

Position yourself in a constructive resting position by lying on your back, legs bent, and feet flat on the ground. Let go of any extra stress in your body by letting it sink into the earth.

• **Pelvic Clock:** Explore the various ranges of mobility by gently rocking your pelvis in a circular manner.

• **Spine Twist:** Take a comfortable seat and gently rotate your body side to side, making sure that each twist lengthens your spine.

• **Arm Circles:** While you slowly and deliberately move your arms in circles, stand tall and pay attention to any feelings in your upper back and shoulders.

The Benefits of Somatic Practice: Engaging in somatic practices may lead to a host of advantages, such as:

Reduced Pain: By addressing underlying muscle imbalances and movement patterns, somatic exercises may assist to reduce chronic pain.

• **Better Posture:** You may naturally align your posture, decreasing strain and increasing optimum performance, by developing a better awareness of your body.

Enhanced Flexibility and Wider Range of Motion: Somatic exercises promote mild muscular stretching and elongation, which increases flexibility.

- **Stress Reduction:** Somatic practice's conscious aspect may aid in nervous system calmness, stress reduction, and relaxation.

- **Greater Body Awareness:** By learning to recognize your body's subtle signals, you'll have a better awareness of your physical self and be more equipped to make decisions that are in line with your wellbeing.

CHAPTER 4: MINDFUL MOVEMENT AND RELAXATION FOR WEIGHT MANAGEMENT

Stress Reduction Techniques: Guided Meditations and Breath work

In our fast-paced world, stress has become an unwelcome companion, casting a shadow over our well-being and hindering our ability to thrive. However, there is a sanctuary of serenity waiting to be discovered—a realm where you can release tension, quiet the mind, and cultivate inner peace. Welcome to the transformative world of guided meditations and breathe work, two powerful tools that can empower you to navigate life's challenges with grace and resilience.

Unveiling the Power of Guided Meditation

Guided meditation is a practice that involves listening to a soothing voice that gently guides you through a series of visualizations, affirmations, or reflections. These carefully crafted narratives transport you to tranquil landscapes, evoke positive emotions, and promote a sense of deep relaxation. By engaging your imagination and focusing your attention, guided meditations can help you:

- **Reduce Stress and Anxiety:** Research has shown that guided meditation can lower cortisol levels, the stress hormone, and activate the parasympathetic nervous system, responsible for rest and relaxation.

- **Improve Sleep Quality:** By calming the mind and body, guided meditation can prepare you for a restful night's sleep.

- **Enhance Emotional Well-being:** Regular practice can cultivate greater self-awareness, compassion, and resilience in the face of life's challenges.

- **Boost Focus and Concentration:** Meditation can train your mind to stay present and focused, improving your cognitive function and productivity.

Discovering the Art of Breath work

Breath work is a conscious manipulation of your breathing patterns to influence your physical, mental, and emotional state. By intentionally controlling your breath, you can tap into its profound healing potential. Breath work exercises can help you:

- **Activate the Relaxation Response:** Deep, diaphragmatic breathing can trigger the relaxation response, a physiological state that counteracts the stress response.

- **Release Tension and Trauma:** Certain breastwork techniques, such as homotopic breastwork, can help to release stored emotions and traumas.

- **Increase Energy and Vitality:** Breath work can oxygenate your body, improve circulation, and boost your energy levels.

- **Enhance Mindfulness and Presence:** By focusing on your breath, you can cultivate greater awareness of the present moment and reduce rumination.

Creating Your Personalized Stress-Reduction Sanctuary

The beauty of guided meditations and breath work lies in their accessibility and versatility. You can practice them anytime, anywhere, and tailor them to your individual needs and preferences. Here's how to create your personalized stress-reduction sanctuary:

1. **Explore Different Styles:** There are countless guided meditations and breath work techniques available. Experiment with different styles to find what resonates with you. Some popular options include mindfulness meditations, body scans, progressive muscle relaxation, alternate nostril breathing, and box breathing.

2. **Find a Quiet Space:** Choose a peaceful environment where you can relax without distractions. Dim the lights, light a candle, or play calming music to enhance the ambiance.

3. **Set an Intention:** Before you begin, take a moment to set an intention for your practice. What do you hope to achieve through meditation or breastwork? Do you want to reduce stress, improve sleep, or simply cultivate inner peace?

4. **Be Patient and Kind:** Meditation and breastwork are skills that take time and practice to master.

Don't get discouraged if your mind wanders or you struggle to focus. Simply bring your attention back to your breath or the guided voice, and continue with kindness and compassion.

5. **Make It a Habit:** To reap the full benefits of these practices, aim to incorporate them into your daily routine. Even a few minutes of meditation or breathwork can make a significant difference in your overall well-being.

Gentle Yoga-Inspired Flows: Promoting Relaxation and Restoration

Escape the hustle and bustle of daily life and immerse yourself in a world of tranquility with gentle yoga-inspired flows. These mindful movements are designed to nurture your body and mind, promoting deep relaxation and restoration. Whether you're a seasoned yogi or a beginner seeking a gentle introduction, these flows offer a sanctuary of calm amidst the chaos.

Unwind and Rejuvenate

Gentle yoga flows are a symphony of slow, deliberate movements that gently stretch and strengthen your muscles, improve flexibility, and release tension. Unlike more vigorous styles of yoga, these flows prioritize fluidity and ease, allowing you to sink deeper into each pose and connect with your breath.

The Benefits of Gentle Yoga Flows

- **Stress Reduction:** The mindful nature of gentle yoga activates the parasympathetic nervous system, responsible for rest and relaxation, helping to reduce stress and anxiety.

- **Improved Sleep:** By calming the mind and body, gentle yoga can prepare you for a restful night's sleep.

- **Pain Relief:** Gentle stretches and movements can alleviate chronic pain, such as back pain, neck pain, and joint stiffness.

- **Enhanced Flexibility and Mobility:** Regular practice can improve your range of motion and flexibility, making everyday activities easier and more enjoyable.

- **Increased Body Awareness:** Gentle yoga encourages you to tune into your body's sensations, fostering a deeper understanding of your physical self.

Creating Your Personalized Gentle Yoga Practice

- **Set the Mood:** Choose a quiet, peaceful space where you can relax without distractions. Dim the lights, light a candle, or play calming music to create a serene atmosphere.

- **Warm Up:** Begin with gentle stretches and movements to prepare your body for deeper poses. Cat-cow pose, child's pose, and seated twists are excellent warm-up options.

- **Flow with Intention:** Choose poses that resonate with your body's needs. Focus on slow, controlled movements, and hold each pose for several breaths, allowing your muscles to release tension.

- **Breathe Deeply:** Your breath is your anchor in gentle yoga. Inhale deeply to expand your chest and belly, and exhale slowly to release tension.

- **Cool Down:** End your practice with a few minutes of relaxation in savasana (corpse pose). Allow your body to completely surrender to the ground as you bask in the afterglow of your practice.

Embrace the Journey of Gentle Yoga

Gentle yoga is a journey of self-discovery and healing. It's an invitation to slow down, listen to your body, and cultivate a deeper connection with yourself. By embracing the gentle flows, you can unlock a world of tranquility and well-being, one breath at a time.

Sample Gentle Yoga Flow:

1. **Child's Pose:** Begin on your hands and knees, then bring your hips back to your heels and rest your forehead on the mat.

2. **Cat-Cow Pose:** Arch your back like a cat on an inhale, then round your back like a cow on an exhale.

3. **Downward-Facing Dog:** From a tabletop position, lift your hips up and back, forming an inverted V-shape with your body.

4. **Warrior II:** Step one foot forward, bend your front knee, and extend your arms out to the sides.

5. **Triangle Pose:** Extend one leg back, hinge at your hips, and reach your hand towards your front foot or the floor.

6. **Savasana:** Lie on your back with your arms at your sides and palms facing up. Close your eyes and relax completely.

Mindful Eating Practices: Cultivating a Healthy Relationship with Food

In a world that often rushes us through meals, rediscover the profound pleasure of eating with mindfulness. Mindful eating is an invitation to slow down, engage your senses, and cultivate a deeper connection with the nourishment that sustains you. It's a transformative practice that can revolutionize your relationship with food, leading to improved digestion, healthier choices, and a greater appreciation for the simple act of eating.

Awaken Your Senses

Mindful eating begins with a sensory awakening. Before you take your first bite, pause to appreciate the visual feast before you. Notice the vibrant colors, the intricate textures, and the enticing aromas that dance in the air. As you bring the food to your mouth, savor the symphony of flavors that unfolds on your palate. Pay attention to the subtle nuances of sweet, salty, sour, and bitter, and allow each bite to linger on your tongue before swallowing.

Tune into Your Body's Wisdom

Mindful eating is not just about savoring flavors; it's also about listening to your body's innate wisdom. As you eat, tune into your hunger and fullness cues. Are you truly hungry, or are you eating out of habit or emotional triggers? Notice the subtle signals your body sends as you eat. Do you feel satisfied, or are you beginning to feel full? By honoring these cues, you can avoid overeating and develop a healthier relationship with food.

Cultivate Gratitude and Appreciation

Mindful eating is an act of gratitude. Take a moment to reflect on the journey your food has taken to reach your plate. Acknowledge the farmers who cultivated the ingredients, the hands that prepared the meal, and the nourishment that it provides for your body and mind. As you eat, express gratitude for the abundance that surrounds you and the pleasure of sharing a meal with loved ones.

Transform Your Eating Experience

Incorporating mindful eating practices into your daily routine can transform your relationship with food. By slowing down, engaging your senses, and honoring your body's wisdom, you can rediscover the joy of eating and cultivate a healthier, more balanced approach to nourishment.

Simple Tips for Mindful Eating:

- **Eliminate Distractions:** Turn off the TV, put away your phone, and create a peaceful environment for your meal.

- **Start Small:** Begin by practicing mindful eating for a few minutes at each meal, gradually increasing the duration as you become more comfortable.

- **Engage Your Senses:** Pay attention to the sights, smells, tastes, textures, and sounds of your food.

- **Chew Thoroughly:** Take your time to chew each bite thoroughly, savoring the flavors and textures.

- **Listen to Your Body:** Pay attention to your hunger and fullness cues, and stop eating when you feel satisfied.

CHAPTER 5: NUTRITION AND SOMATIC EXERCISE: A HOLISTIC APPROACH

Eating for Energy and Weight Loss: The Somatic Nutrition Principles

Tired of restrictive diets that leave you feeling deprived and drained? Craving a sustainable approach to weight loss that nourishes your body and mind? Look no further than the transformative power of Somatic Nutrition. This revolutionary approach to eating transcends mere calorie counting and restrictive meal plans, inviting you to embark on a journey of self-discovery, intuitive eating, and sustainable weight management.

The Essence of Somatic Nutrition

Somatic Nutrition is a holistic approach that honors the intricate connection between your body, mind, and the food you consume. It goes beyond simply what you eat, delving into the how and why of your eating habits. By cultivating body awareness, mindful eating practices, and a deep understanding of your individual needs, you can unlock a profound transformation in your relationship with food and your body.

The Principles of Somatic Nutrition

1. **Honor Your Hunger:** Listen to your body's innate signals of hunger and fullness. Eat when you're truly hungry, and stop when you're comfortably satisfied.

2. **Savor Each Bite:** Engage all your senses as you eat. Notice the colors, aromas, textures, and flavors of your food. Chew slowly and savor each bite, allowing your body to fully digest and absorb the nutrients.

3. **Embrace Pleasure:** Food is meant to be enjoyed! Choose foods that nourish your body and delight your taste buds. Allow yourself to indulge in moderation, without guilt or shame.

4. **Nourish Your Body:** Prioritize whole, unprocessed foods that provide your body with the nutrients it needs to thrive. Focus on colorful fruits and vegetables, lean protein, healthy fats, and whole grains.

5. **Listen to Your Body's Wisdom:** Your body is constantly communicating with you. Pay attention to how different foods make you feel. Notice if certain foods trigger digestive discomfort, fatigue, or mood swings. Use this information to make informed choices that support your well-being.

The Transformative Power of Somatic Nutrition

By embracing the principles of Somatic Nutrition, you can:

- **Achieve Sustainable Weight Loss:** By listening to your body's signals and choosing nourishing foods, you can naturally regulate your appetite and achieve a healthy weight without deprivation.

- **Boost Energy Levels:** Whole, unprocessed foods provide your body with sustained energy, eliminating the crashes and cravings associated with processed foods and sugar.

- **Improve Digestion:** Mindful eating and a focus on whole foods can promote optimal digestion and reduce digestive discomfort.

- **Enhance Mood and Well-being:** Nourishing your body with wholesome foods can positively impact your mood, reduce anxiety, and improve overall well-being.

- **Cultivate a Positive Relationship with Food:** Somatic Nutrition empowers you to break free from restrictive dieting and develop a healthy, sustainable relationship with food.

Mindful Eating in Practice: Tips and Techniques for Success

guide to Mastering Mindful Eating

Ready to transform your relationship with food and embark on a culinary adventure that nourishes your body and soul? Mindful eating is your passport to a more satisfying, healthier, and joyful eating experience. Let's delve into the practical tips and techniques that will empower you to savor each bite and unlock the full potential of this transformative practice.

Set the Stage for Mindful Eating

- **Create a Sacred Space:** Designate a calm and inviting eating area, free from distractions like screens and clutter. Light a candle, play soft music, or arrange a simple table setting to enhance the ambiance.

- **Engage Your Senses:** Before taking your first bite, pause to admire the vibrant colors, inhale the enticing aromas, and appreciate the textures of your meal. This sensory exploration sets the stage for a more mindful experience.

- **Start Small:** Begin by practicing mindful eating with one meal a day. As you become more comfortable, gradually incorporate it into all your meals and snacks.

During Your Mindful Meal

- **Chew Thoroughly:** Slow down and savor each bite. Aim to chew each mouthful at least 20-30 times before swallowing. This aids digestion and allows you to fully appreciate the flavors.

- **Tune into Your Body:** Pay close attention to your hunger and fullness cues. Eat when you're truly hungry, and stop when you feel comfortably satisfied, not overly full.

- **Appreciate the Journey:** Reflect on the origins of your food and the effort that went into its creation. Express gratitude for the nourishment it provides.

- **Avoid Multitasking:** Resist the urge to scroll through your phone, watch TV, or read while eating. Focus solely on the present moment and the experience of eating.

Overcoming Challenges

- **Emotional Eating:** If you find yourself reaching for food in response to emotions, pause and explore alternative coping mechanisms, such as journaling, talking to a friend, or going for a walk.

- **Social Eating:** When dining with others, be present in the conversation and enjoy the company. However, don't feel pressured to eat at the same pace as others. Listen to your body's signals and eat at a comfortable pace.

- **Cravings:** Cravings are a natural part of life. Instead of suppressing them, acknowledge them with curiosity. Take a few deep breaths, explore the craving mindfully, and then decide whether to indulge in moderation or choose a healthier alternative.

The Rewards of Mindful Eating

The benefits of mindful eating extend far beyond the dining table. By practicing mindful eating, you can:

- **Improve Digestion:** Slowing down and chewing thoroughly aids digestion and reduces digestive discomfort.

- **Manage Weight:** By tuning into your body's hunger and fullness cues, you can avoid overeating and make healthier food choices.

- **Reduce Stress:** Mindful eating promotes relaxation and reduces stress by activating the parasympathetic nervous system.

- **Enhance Enjoyment of Food:** By savoring each bite, you can fully appreciate the flavors, textures, and aromas of your food.

- **Cultivate a Healthier Relationship with Food:** Mindful eating can help you break free from emotional eating patterns and develop a more positive relationship with food.

Sample Meal Plans and Recipes: Delicious and Nourishing Options

Ready to tantalize your taste buds and nourish your body with delicious, mindful meals? This curated collection of sample meal plans and recipes will ignite your culinary creativity and inspire you to embrace a more conscious approach to eating. Each dish is crafted with wholesome ingredients, vibrant flavors, and a touch of mindfulness, ensuring a truly satisfying and nourishing experience.

Energizing Breakfast Options

- **Mindful Morning Smoothie:** Blend together a symphony of flavors with spinach, banana, berries, Greek yogurt, and a sprinkle of chia seeds. Sip slowly, savoring each sip and appreciating the burst of nutrients.

- **Savory Oatmeal with Poached Egg:** Elevate your oatmeal game with a poached egg nestled atop a bed of creamy oats cooked in almond milk. Sprinkle with chopped herbs, a drizzle of olive oil, and a pinch of sea salt for a savory and satisfying breakfast.

- **Avocado Toast with a Twist:** Toast a slice of whole-grain bread and top it with creamy avocado, a sprinkle of feta cheese, a drizzle of balsamic glaze, and a sprinkle of red pepper flakes for a delightful combination of textures and flavors.

Nourishing Lunch Delights

- **Mediterranean Quinoa Salad:** Embrace the vibrant flavors of the Mediterranean with this quinoa salad bursting with cucumbers, tomatoes, Kalamata olives, feta cheese, and a zesty lemon-herb vinaigrette.

- **Lentil Soup with Turmeric and Ginger:** Warm your soul with a comforting bowl of lentil soup infused with the anti-inflammatory properties of turmeric and ginger. Add a dollop of coconut milk for extra creaminess and a sprinkle of cilantro for a touch of freshness.

- **Turkey Lettuce Wraps:** Ditch the tortillas and wrap your favorite fillings in crisp lettuce leaves. Combine ground turkey, shredded carrots, diced cucumbers, and a drizzle of peanut sauce for a light and refreshing lunch.

Satisfying Dinner Creations

- **Salmon with Roasted Vegetables:** Bake a succulent salmon fillet seasoned with herbs and spices alongside a colorful medley of roasted vegetables, such as broccoli, carrots, and Brussels sprouts. Drizzle with a balsamic glaze for a touch of sweetness.

- **Chicken Stir-Fry with Brown Rice:** Whip up a quick and flavorful stir-fry with chicken, broccoli, bell peppers, and snap peas. Serve over brown rice and drizzle with a savory sauce made with soy sauce, ginger, and garlic.

- **Vegetarian Chili:** Embrace the hearty goodness of vegetarian chili packed with beans, corn, tomatoes, and a blend of warming spices. Top with avocado, shredded cheese, and a dollop of Greek yogurt for a complete and satisfying meal.

Mindful Snacking

- **Greek Yogurt with Berries and Nuts:** Enjoy a creamy and satisfying snack with Greek yogurt topped with a handful of mixed berries and a sprinkle of chopped nuts.

- **Carrot Sticks with Hummus:** Dip crunchy carrot sticks into a creamy hummus for a healthy and flavorful snack.

- **Hard-Boiled Egg with Avocado:** Combine protein and healthy fats with a hard-boiled egg and half an avocado, seasoned with salt and pepper.

CHAPTER 6: LIFESTYLE HABITS FOR LONG-TERM WEIGHT MANAGEMENT SUCCESS

Sleep: The Essential Ingredient for Weight Loss and Overall Health

Power of Sleep

In our relentless pursuit of well-being, we often overlook a fundamental pillar of health that holds the key to unlocking our full potential: sleep. Far beyond mere rest, sleep is a dynamic process that orchestrates a symphony of physiological functions crucial for weight management and overall vitality. Let's delve into the intricate relationship between sleep and weight loss, exploring how prioritizing quality slumber can revolutionize your journey to a healthier, happier you.

Sleep: The Unsung Hero of Weight Loss

While diet and exercise often steal the spotlight in weight loss discussions, sleep plays a pivotal role in achieving and maintaining a healthy weight. When we sleep, our bodies engage in a complex interplay of hormonal regulation, energy balance, and metabolic processes that directly impact our weight. Research has consistently shown that insufficient sleep can disrupt these delicate mechanisms, leading to weight gain and hindering weight loss efforts.

The Hormonal Dance: Ghrelin and Leptin

Two key hormones, ghrelin and leptin, play a crucial role in regulating our appetite and satiety. Ghrelin, the "hunger hormone," stimulates appetite, while leptin, the "satiety hormone," signals fullness. Sleep deprivation disrupts the delicate balance of these hormones, leading to increased ghrelin levels, heightened cravings, and decreased leptin levels, making us feel less satisfied after meals. This hormonal imbalance can trigger overeating and sabotage our weight loss goals.

The Metabolic Symphony: Energy Expenditure and Glucose Regulation

Sleep deprivation not only affects our appetite hormones but also disrupts our metabolism. Studies have shown that insufficient sleep can decrease resting metabolic rate, the number of calories we burn at rest, and impair glucose regulation, leading to insulin resistance. These metabolic disruptions can hinder fat burning and promote fat storage, making weight loss more challenging.

The Mind-Body Connection: Stress, Cravings, and Decision-Making

Sleep deprivation not only takes a toll on our physical health but also impacts our mental and emotional well-being. Lack of sleep can increase stress levels, which in turn can trigger cravings for unhealthy foods and impair our ability to make sound decisions. This vicious cycle can lead to unhealthy eating habits and hinder weight loss progress.

Prioritize Sleep, Optimize Health

To harness the transformative power of sleep for weight loss and overall health, make sleep a non-negotiable priority in your life. Aim for 7-8 hours of quality sleep each night, establish a consistent sleep schedule, create a relaxing bedtime routine, and optimize your sleep environment for darkness, quiet, and comfort.

The Rewards of Restful Slumber

Investing in quality sleep is an investment in your health and well-being. By prioritizing sleep, you can:

- **Achieve and Maintain a Healthy Weight:** Regulate appetite hormones, optimize metabolism, and reduce cravings for unhealthy foods.

- **Boost Energy Levels:** Wake up feeling refreshed, energized, and ready to tackle the day.

- **Enhance Mood and Cognitive Function:** Improve focus, concentration, and decision-making abilities.

- **Strengthen Immunity:** Support your body's natural defenses against illness and disease.

- **Reduce Stress and Improve Overall Well-being:** Promote relaxation, reduce anxiety, and enhance your overall quality of life.

Stress Management: Strategies for Reducing Stress and Emotional Eating

Are stress and emotional eating hijacking your well-being? Imagine reclaiming control, feeling calmer, and making empowered choices about food. It's entirely possible with a toolbox of effective stress management strategies designed to nurture your mind, body, and spirit.

Unmasking Emotional Eating

Emotional eating is a common coping mechanism, often triggered by stress, anxiety, boredom, or sadness. It can lead to a vicious cycle of guilt and shame, further fueling stress levels. Recognizing these triggers is the first step towards breaking free. Ask yourself: Am I truly hungry, or am I seeking comfort?

Stress-Busting Strategies

1. **Mindful Movement:** Engage in activities that get you moving and reconnect you with your body. Yoga, tai chi, dance, or even a brisk walk can release endorphins, the body's natural mood boosters, and alleviate stress.

2. **Breathe Deeply:** When stress strikes, pause and take a few deep breaths. Inhale slowly and deeply, filling your belly with air, then exhale slowly. This simple act can activate the relaxation response, calming your nervous system.

3. **Cultivate Mindfulness:** Practice mindfulness meditation to anchor yourself in the present moment. Observe your thoughts and feelings without judgment, allowing them to come and go like passing clouds. This can help you become more aware of emotional triggers and create space for healthier responses.

4. **Connect with Nature:** Spending time in nature has a profound calming effect. Immerse yourself in the

sights, sounds, and smells of the outdoors. Go for a hike, sit by a lake, or simply stroll through a park.

5. **Prioritize Sleep:** Quality sleep is essential for stress management and overall well-being. Aim for 7-8 hours of restful sleep each night to allow your body and mind to recharge.

6. **Nurture Supportive Relationships:** Connect with loved ones who uplift and support you. Share your struggles and seek their encouragement.

Alternative Coping Mechanisms

- **Journaling:** Write down your thoughts and feelings to gain clarity and release pent-up emotions.

- **Creative Expression:** Engage in activities that spark joy and creativity, such as painting, drawing, writing, or playing music.

- **Self-Care Rituals:** Take time for yourself each day to relax and recharge. This could involve taking a warm bath, reading a book, or simply enjoying a cup of tea.

Mindful Eating Tips

- **Pause before You Eat:** Take a few moments to check in with your hunger levels. Are you truly hungry, or are you eating for another reason?

- **Savor Each Bite:** Engage all your senses as you eat. Notice the flavors, textures, and aromas of your food. Chew slowly and savor each bite.

- **Choose Nourishing Foods:** Opt for whole, unprocessed foods that fuel your body and mind. Avoid sugary drinks and processed snacks, which can lead to energy crashes and mood swings.

- **Hydrate:** Drink plenty of water throughout the day to stay hydrated and curb cravings.

Seeking Support

If you're struggling to manage stress and emotional eating on your own, don't hesitate to seek professional help. A therapist or counselor can provide guidance and support to help you develop healthy coping mechanisms and break free from the cycle of emotional eating.

Creating a Supportive Environment: Building a Foundation for Success

Imagine stepping into a space where your dreams feel not just possible, but inevitable. A space where you are celebrated, challenged, and empowered to reach your full potential. This is the transformative power of a supportive environment—a fertile ground where seeds of ambition blossom into extraordinary achievements. Let's delve into the art of cultivating such an environment, a sanctuary that nurtures your growth and propels you towards unparalleled success.

The Pillars of a Supportive Environment

1. **Unwavering Belief:** At the heart of any supportive environment lies an unwavering belief in your abilities. Surround yourself with individuals who champion your dreams, who see your potential even when you doubt yourself, and who offer encouragement and constructive feedback.

2. **Nurturing Relationships:** Forge genuine connections with people who inspire, uplift, and challenge you. Seek mentors who have walked the

path before you, peers who share your passions, and collaborators who bring diverse perspectives to the table.

3. **Open Communication:** Foster a culture of open and honest communication, where ideas flow freely, feedback is welcomed, and conflicts are resolved constructively. Create safe spaces for dialogue, where everyone feels heard, valued, and respected.

4. **Positive Reinforcement:** Celebrate both big and small wins, recognizing the effort and dedication that goes into every step of your journey. Positive reinforcement fuels motivation, builds confidence, and reinforces a growth mindset.

5. **Growth Mindset:** Embrace challenges as opportunities for learning and development. View setbacks as temporary roadblocks, not permanent failures. Cultivate a resilience that allows you to bounce back stronger and wiser from every experience.

Creating Your Supportive Ecosystem

- **Choose Your Circle Wisely:** Surround yourself with individuals who align with your values, who inspire you to be your best self, and who support your aspirations.

- **Set Clear Boundaries** :Protect your energy and focus by setting boundaries with individuals who drain or discourage you.

- **Invest in Personal Development:** Continuously seek knowledge, acquire new skills, and expand your horizons. Attend workshops, read books, listen to podcasts, and engage in activities that challenge and inspire you.

- **Practice Self-Care:** Prioritize your physical, mental, and emotional well-being. Engage in activities that nourish your soul, reduce stress, and recharge your batteries.

- **Embrace Community:** Join or create communities of like-minded individuals who share your passions and goals. The collective energy and support of a community can be a powerful catalyst for growth.

The Ripple Effect of a Supportive Environment

A supportive environment not only benefits you as an individual but also radiates outward, positively impacting those around you. By fostering a culture of encouragement, collaboration, and growth, you create a ripple effect that inspires others to reach their full potential.

PART IV: INSPIRATION AND RESOURCES

CHAPTER 7: SUCCESS STORIES: REAL PEOPLE, REAL TRANSFORMATIONS

Inspiring Stories of Weight Loss through Somatic Exercise: Finding Motivation

Tired of fad diets and grueling workouts? Discover the inspiring journeys of individuals who have shed pounds and reclaimed their vitality through the gentle power of somatic exercise. These stories are a testament to the profound connection between mind and body, showcasing how mindful movement can transform not only your physique but also your relationship with yourself.

Meet Sarah, who struggled with chronic back pain and emotional eating. Through somatic practices, she not only shed excess weight but also found solace and empowerment. Join John, a former athlete sidelined by injuries, who rediscovered the joy of movement and regained his strength through gentle, mindful exercise. These are just a few examples of the countless lives touched by somatic exercise.

If you're seeking a sustainable path to weight loss that nourishes your body and soul, let these stories ignite your motivation. Embrace the transformative power of somatic exercise and embark on your own journey to a healthier, happier you.

The path to weight loss, much like life itself, is seldom a smooth, linear trajectory. It's a journey peppered with challenges, plateaus, and moments of self-doubt. Yet, within these obstacles lie invaluable lessons and opportunities for growth. Let's delve into the inspiring stories of individuals who have navigated the twists and turns of somatic weight loss, emerging stronger, wiser, and more empowered than ever before.

Meet Emily: A mother of two who struggled with years of yo-yo dieting and negative body image. Through somatic practices, she learned to listen to her body's cues, cultivate self-compassion, and break free from the cycle of restrictive eating. Emily's journey reminds us that weight loss is not a race but a lifelong process of self-discovery and self-acceptance.

David's Story: A former athlete plagued by chronic injuries, David found solace in somatic movement. He discovered that gentle, mindful exercise could not only alleviate his pain but also reignite his passion for movement. David's story teaches us the importance of adapting our approach to exercise as our bodies evolve and embracing the healing power of mindful movement.

Maria's Transformation: Maria, a busy professional, struggled with stress-induced weight gain and emotional eating. Through somatic practices, she learned to identify her triggers, manage stress, and cultivate a healthier relationship with food. Maria's journey highlights the profound impact that stress management and emotional well-being have on our weight loss efforts.

Lessons Learned, Wisdom Gained

These inspiring stories offer valuable lessons for anyone navigating the challenges and plateaus of weight loss:

- **Patience is a Virtue:** Weight loss is not an overnight process. Embrace the journey, celebrate small victories, and trust that consistent effort will yield results.

- **Listen to Your Body:** Your body is your wisest guide. Pay attention to its signals of hunger, fullness, and energy levels. Honor your body's unique needs and adjust your approach accordingly.

- **Embrace Self-Compassion:** Be kind to yourself, especially during setbacks and plateaus. Remember that progress is not always linear, and setbacks are a natural part of the journey.

- **Seek Support:** Surround yourself with a supportive community of like-minded individuals who can offer encouragement, guidance, and accountability.

- **Celebrate Your Wins:** Acknowledge your achievements, no matter how small they may seem. Celebrate each milestone as a testament to your dedication and resilience.

CONCLUSION

As you close the final pages of this book, a new chapter in your wellness journey begins. You've delved into the depths of somatic exercise, discovering its remarkable potential to transform not only your body but also your mind and spirit. You've learned how to listen to your body's wisdom, cultivate mindful movement, and nourish yourself with intention. You've explored the profound connection between stress, emotions, and weight, and armed yourself with powerful tools to overcome challenges and plateaus.

Now, it's time to step into the world with renewed confidence, empowered by the knowledge and practices you've gained. Let the principles of somatic exercise guide you as you navigate the path to sustainable weight loss and vibrant health. Remember, this is not a destination but a lifelong journey of self-discovery, growth, and transformation.

Embrace the gentle power of movement, savor the joy of nourishing your body, and cultivate a deep appreciation for the interconnectedness of your physical, mental, and emotional well-being. Let somatic exercise be your compass, guiding you towards a life of vitality, balance, and radiant health.

As you continue on this path, remember that you are not alone. Surround yourself with a supportive community, share your experiences, and celebrate your victories. Let the collective wisdom and encouragement of others fuel your motivation and inspire you to reach new heights.

The journey to a healthier, happier you starts with a single step. Take that step today, and embrace the transformative power of somatic exercise. Your body, mind, and spirit will thank you.

A Heartfelt Thank You

Thank you for embarking on this somatic journey with me. It has been an honor to share my knowledge and experience with you. I hope this book has inspired you to embrace a more mindful, holistic approach to weight loss and well-being.

If you found this book valuable and insightful, I would be deeply grateful if you would **consider leaving a 5-star**

review. **Your feedback is invaluable to me, and it helps
others discover** the transformative power of somatic
exercise.